Health Is For Everyone

Heart Problems?
Stop: The Pain, Suffering & Early
Death Causes & Solutions Revealed

Frederick Mickel Huck

authorHOUSE®

AuthorHouse™
1663 Liberty Drive
Bloomington, IN 47403
www.authorhouse.com
Phone: 1-800-839-8640

First published by AuthorHouse 1/4/2010

ISBN: 978-1-4490-5308-6 (sc)

Library of Congress Control Number: 2009912492

Printed in the United States of America
Bloomington, Indiana

This book is printed on acid-free paper.

This book is dedicated to:

ROBERT E MENZIE

INEZ A MENZIE

DONALD W HUCK

AURA V HUCK

DR EDE KOENIG

Special thanks to:

SANDRA V MOONEY

MATTHEW F MOONEY

JOHN DUNLAP

ANGIE INGERSOLL

The Causes of Heart Problems

Heart disease is the number one killer of human beings in the United States. To the surprise of many, it is not cancer. The medical system of the United States as we know it, only treats the symptoms of heart disease, but not the causes. Heart disease causes pain and suffering, many expensive trips to the doctors, and hospitals, and the use of many expensive medications that have horrible side effects and the result is usually death.

Many popular drugs like coumadin are a form of poison, which has side effects like high blood pressure. In fact, coumadin is often used in rat poison. Another drug of choice that the medical industry uses on heart disease is nitro glycerin for angina. If you care about your body and your well-being, you should not subject it to that poison. It is a fact that all strokes are caused by a blood clot in the brain that stops the flow of oxygen being pumped throughout the brain. If a person is given nitroglycerin, it can cause a blood clot to form in the brain and can lead to a stroke and possibly death.

Do Not Blame The Animals

Animals or animal products do not belong in the human body; they do not mix and are carcinogenic, toxic, and full of bacteria, parasites, worms, and chemicals. Pork products are packed in sulfa. Nitro furans are found in poultry and large amounts of antibiotics are found in beef, poultry and pork. In fact, more than forty per cent of all antibiotics that are manufactured are placed in meat products and are a recipe for chemical contamination. Meat meant for human consumption contains cancer viruses, blood, mold, pollutants, allergies, and uric acid. Meat products have more measurable amounts of bacteria than fresh manure. It is a fact! Meat also has hormones, saturated fat, cholesterol, and chemicals that cause the meat to have a better color for cosmetic purposes, and to mask the appearance of diseased and mistreated animals. Meat can easily be preserved for months and even years before being consumed. The meat industry is currently fighting disclosure of information about the marketing of meat with well-paid lobbyists. It is not advantageous for the meat industry for the consumer to know how long an animal has been dead, rotting, and decaying. The longer between the death of the animal and its consumption, the more parasites, worms, and bacteria are present. The meat industry knows that the customer would be less likely to buy meat if the industry had to disclose this information to the customer and their profits would most likely fall. It is an indisputable fact science has learned how to package animal products that have mold or a rotten smell; and make the products appear fresh. All products that contain animal parts, including animal blood, spoil or rot when the animal is killed. It is a fact of nature. Modern science along with pharmaceutical and chemical industries have found a way to slow down this natural process and the consumer is now eating these chemicals, which do not contain any nutrition; but contains toxins. It is estimated that only one person out of a hundred will continue to eat meat if they witness how animals are prepared for human consumption. Animals consume at least seventy percent of all grains produced in the United States. A large amount of the forests in the United States is used each year by the meat industry. In Brazil, the raising of animals causes fifty percent of the rain forest destruction. Animals that are raised to be eaten will drink two to three thousand gallons of water for each pound of meat that will be produced. The animal waste pollutes the human water supply, land and environment. In fact, the world's meat production contributes more to pollution and greenhouse effects than industry. The meat industry makes for an imbalance of nature and is inhumanly cruel to the way it treats animals. It is difficult to view this madness without the feeling of despair and revolation.

Facts About Meat

The numbers tell the story of another cause of preventable strokes and that is the consumption of meat. Lung functions are significantly decreased, up to forty-eight hours after the consumption of meats, which means less oxygen gets into the blood, blood pressure rises, and the potential for blood clots increase. The risk of ovarian, colon, prostate cancer, arthritis, osteoporosis, kidney and gallstones increase significantly when a person consumes meat. It is scientifically and statistically proven that in comparing countries that do not consume meat, that heart problems are rare as compared to the United States and other developed countries who consume high amounts of meat. In addition, meat has no fiber and is an incomplete source of nutrition. It is estimated that in the United States the average meat eater will consume in their lifetime the following: * 10 to 15 thousand chickens * 15 to 20 cows * about 2000 fish * 24 to 34 pigs * 12 to 15 sheep * Mankind was not designed to be meat or flesh eaters as demonstrated by the mouth and teeth. Humans were designed to be fruit, vegetable, nut, and grain eaters. Each year many people suffer from what they think is the flu, but it is actually from eating contaminated animal products. Diseases like salmonella, staphylococcus, and psittacosis, all are transmitted from animal to humans. The strongest animals in the world are the elephant (who can live to be 100 years old), the water buffalo, camels, mules, and horses. These animals have one thing in common they are all vegetarian eaters. Lions that eat meat sleep around 20 hours a day. Cats and dogs live about 15 years, eat mainly meat but have large amounts of uric acid. They have a mouth and teeth meant for eating meat. Humans on the other hand do not have mouths to eat meat and their mouths are meant to be fruit, vegetable, nuts and grain eaters.

Notes From The Author

The definition of the word "food" as I understand is something that when consumed, nourishes the human body without causing unhealthy side effects. Poison is not food, as it will lead to a slow or fast death. Therefore, when the reader of the book reads the words "no food" or "fake food" it strictly that it means to convey a type of poison as it does not nourish the human body.

Fourteen Days Guide

The purpose of this fourteen-day meal plan is to illustrate that starvation does not exist when following the plan. Instead of listing the fruit on a daily log everyday, I just list here approximately, what was eaten. For the last two years, I have reversed my two meals. The larger was consumed first and the second is mostly raw. Prior to eating breakfast, generally a half an hour after I wake, I drink a quart of warm water with two teaspoons of lemon juice, one tablespoon of inland sea water, and one tablespoon of silver mineral water. I consume approximately five pounds of fruit daily and the fruit varies according to the seasons of the year. The fourteen days are very similar (fruit meal) and they are three different colors of apples, twelve cherries, one nectarine, one mango, one slice of pineapple, one slice of cantaloupe, eight green grapes, one apricot, and one peach. In addition, I also eat eight raw Brazil nuts, six apricot nuts, one teaspoon of sunflower seeds, one teaspoon of pumpkin seeds, two capsules of calcium, and two capsules of magnesium. For dinner, I usually have a salad that consists of red or green head lettuce, three radishes cut small, and one long green onion cut small. In addition, one third of a carrot cut small, one half of avocado, and one half of celery stalk cut small. I complete my dinner with six tablespoons of lemon juice approximately, one tablespoon or more of Braggs Ammino, and up to twelve ounces or more of two different kinds of Hot Sauce, with bread, crackers, or corn tortillas.

Please do not copy or give away any material, not just because it is copyright protected material, but doing this will interfere with my program of feeding and educating the unhealthy. All book proceeds as of 2008 have gone into this program. Instead, my wish is that you do share your cooking with friends, family, and strangers.

Questions, concerns, and suggestions are welcome:

7619 N "8th" St
Fresno, CA 93720-2644
Phone   559 435 4069

14 Days of Meals

Day 1

Breakfast: Fruit,

Raw nuts,

6 ounces of Havanero dry roasted nut mix

Dinner: Salad,

bread,

doubles baked spicy potatoes,

6 ounces of bell pepper rice.

Dessert: Walnut pie

Notes: _____

_____

_____

Day 2

Breakfast: Fruit,

Raw nuts,

cashew waffles

Dinner: Salad,

Corn Tortillas; Roast,

6 ounces of Black eye pea rice

Dessert: Cinnamon Sucanat Sugar cookies

Notes: _____

_____

_____

Day 3

Breakfast: Fruit,

Raw nuts,

two pieces of whole-wheat toast with pineapple jam

Dinner: Salad,

crackers,

Bell Peppers,

Spanish rice

Dessert: Walnut peppermint fudge

Notes: _____

_____

_____

Day 4

Breakfast: Fruit,

                Raw nuts,

                Bell Pepper Rice

Dinner: Salad,

                12 ounces of Lentils,

                12 ounces of Baked Brown Rice

Dessert: Lemon ice cream, 6 ounces

Notes: _____

           _____

           _____

Day 5

Breakfast: Fruit,

Raw nuts,

Bowl of baked oatmeal

Dinner: Salad,

bread,

12 ounces of Black bean soup,

12 ounces of Cajon rice

Dessert: One fourth pound of Peppermint Carmel Candy

Notes: _____

_____

_____

Day 6

Breakfast: Fruit,

                Raw nuts,

                6 ounces Garlic Dry Roasted Nut mix

Dinner: Salad,

                bread,

                tomato casserole

Dessert: One fourth pound of Coconut cake

Notes: _____

                _____

                _____

Day 7

Breakfast: Fruit,

Raw nuts,

Tofu pancakes

Dinner: Bread,

Taco salad

Dessert: One fourth pound R H I coconut cookies

Notes: _____

_____

_____

Day 8

Breakfast: Fruit,

Raw nuts,

Spanish rice

Dinner: Salad,

crackers,

Pot pie

Dessert: One fourth pound of Roma Dome Cookies

Notes: _____

_____

_____

Day 9

Breakfast: Fruit,

Raw nuts,

cashew waffles

Dinner: Salad,

bread,

Enchiladas

Dessert: One fourth pound of Pecan Fudge

Notes: _____

_____

_____

Day 10

Breakfast: Fruit,

Raw nuts,

Cajon nut mix

Dinner: Salad,

crackers,

Chinese soup,

Chinese rice

Dessert: Raisin cup cookies

Notes: _____

_____

_____

Day 11

Breakfast: Fruit,

Raw nuts,

Bowl of Popcorn

Dinner: Salad,

bread,

Egg Rolls

Dessert: Carob Ice cream

Notes: _____
_____
_____

Day 12

Breakfast: Fruit,

Raw nuts,

two pieces of toast with Peach jam

Dinner: Salad,

bread,

Pasta

Dessert: One fourth pound of Carob salt water taffy

Notes: _____

_____

_____

Day 13

Breakfast: Fruit,

Raw nuts,

Havanero Rice

Dinner: Salad,

corn tortillas,

Pocket Pizzas

Dessert: One fourth pound of Carob Brownies

Notes: _____

_____

_____

Day 14

Breakfast: Fruit,

              Raw nuts,

              Pistachio waffles

Dinner: Salad,

            soymilk cornbread,

            black eye peas,

            garlic and herbs baked rice.

Dessert: Plum Baked Alaska

Notes: _____

            _____

            _____

Setting Up The Pantry

CELL FOOD

1 -800 - 749 - 9196

www.luminahealth.com

Lemon Powder Star West Botanicals

www.starwestbotanicals.com

100% natural ingredients

Air Therapy Purification Mist

www.miarose.com 1-800-292-6339

Wheat Germ- Raw only high source of Vitamin E

Seventh Generation Household Products

www.seventhgeneration.com 1 - 800-456 -1191

Dish liquid and other products

Maria Trebens Authentic Swedish Bitters - no alcohol

110 Bismark St., Concordia, Mo. 64020

Recipe 170

WHIPPED CREAM

In a small pan, place the following:

> One cup soymilk
> One fourth teaspoon rose water
> One fourth teaspoon Biosalt
> Two Tablespoons tapioca

Boil in pan for 2 - 5 minutes and stir.

Then place the above in a vitamix or blender.

Pour into bowl and add One cup coconut flour.

This is not sweet.

Place any doughnut frosting under whipped cream

Notes: _____

_____

_____

Recipe 171

COCONUT CREAM TOPPING # 1

Place the following in a vitamix:

    One cup oatmeal
    Three fourths cup coconut flour
    One cup water
    One fourth teaspoon Biosalt
    One fourth teaspoon vanilla
    One cup maple syrup

Continue to blend until smooth

Place in refrigerator

Notes: _____
_____
_____

Recipe 172

COCONUT CREAM TOPPING

Place the following in a vitamix:

    Two cups oatmeal flour
    One and half cups coconut flour
    2 to 3 and a half cups water
    One fourth to one half teaspoon Biosalt
    One fourth teaspoon vanilla

Continue to blend and refrigerate

This is not sweet; do not put too much on top anything

Can add a color

See color recipe # 193. (This is for decoration only)

Notes: _____

Recipe 173

MOHAMAD TATHI MALEK CAROB MOUSSE

Place in a vitamix the following:

 4 tablespoons tapioca
 One cup sucanant sugar
 One fourth cup cashews
 One fourth cup carob
 One half cup maple syrup
 One tablespoon roma
 One half teaspoon lemon juice
 One brick or One pound tofu
 One fourth teaspoon Biosalt

Continue to blend until ingredients are smooth.

Serve chilled

Notes: _____
 _____
 _____

Recipe 174

CATSUP No. 1

Place in a vitamix the following:

    Three fourths cup tomato paste
    One tablespoon maple syrup
    One tablespoon lemon juice
    One half teaspoon Biosalt
    One half teaspoon onion powder
    One fourth teaspoon garlic powder
    One half teaspoon oregano

Mix until smooth, can freeze extra until ready to use

Notes: _____

_____

_____

Recipe 175 —————————————————————————

ALMOND CAROB ROMA CANDY

Place the following in a vitamix:

> One fourth cup soymilk and Two tablespoons soymilk
> One fourth cup pineapple juice and Two tablespoons pineapple juice
> One fourth teaspoon Biosalt
> Two thirds cup almond butter
> Two cups maple syrup
> One teaspoon rosewater
> One third cup carob powder
> One third cup roma powder, then pour into a large bowl and add
> Two cups coconut

Mix all ingredients. Pour into a glass dish (7 X 7 inches) lined with parchment paper. Then add One cup roasted almonds on top. Place in freezer

Cut into squares, just before serving

Notes: ——————————————————————————
——————————————————————————
——————————————————————————

Recipe 176

ANGEL MACROONS

In a large bowl places the following:

    One cup maple syrup
    One and a half cups dried pineapple or dried papaya (cut small)
    100 roasted almonds (chopped)

Mix by hand and set aside:

Place the following in a vitamix on high until it becomes a liquid, add 9 cups coconut. After 9 cups coconut are liquid, pour into the large bowl and mix by hand with the above. Place on a cookie tray lined with parchment paper, or a cookie mat. Form into shape, then place in the refrigerator

Notes: _____

_____

_____

Recipe 177 ————————————————————

NUT MILK

Place the following: in a vitamix or blender:

    One fourth cup sunflower seeds
    One fourth cup almonds
    One fourth teaspoon Biosalt
    Four cups water
    One fourth cup maple syrup

Continue to blend until all ingredients are liquid

Notes: ————————————————————
————————————————————
————————————————————

Recipe 178

ROMA PIE

Place in a vitamix the following:

>   One half cup boiling water
>   One half cup tapioca
>   One tablespoon tapioca

Then add:

>   One brick or One pound tofu
>   Two cups maple syrup
>   One fourth teaspoon Biosalt
>   One cup roma

Continue to blend until ingredients are smooth.

For pie shell crust, see special piecrust recipe # 38

Can put coconut on top

Notes: _____

_____

_____

Recipe 179

MUSTARD SPREAD

Place the following: in a vitamix or blender:

    One half cup cashews

    Two thirds cup water

    One half teaspoon Biosalt

    Two teaspoons turmeric powder

    8 tablespoons lemon juice

    One fourth teaspoon onion powder

    One eighth teaspoon garlic powder

    One fourth teaspoon paprika

    One fourth teaspoon carob

Continue to blend until ingredients are smooth, then pour into a small pan and boil and stir until thickened.

Can freeze extra until needed

Notes: _____

_____

_____

Recipe 180

CAROB ROMA FROSTING

Place the following: in a vitamix or blender:

    Two cups sucanant sugar
    Two cups maple syrup
    One cup carob
    One cup roma
    8 tablespoons almond butter

Mix, can add to cookies or cakes

Notes: _____

_____

_____

Recipe 181

BASIC FROSTING

Place the following: in a vitamix or blender:

>   One cup soymilk
>   5 tablespoons whole-wheat pastry flour
>   One cup almond butter
>   One cup maple syrup
>   One teaspoon rosewater

Can add One tablespoon each carob or roma (Pero)

Notes: _____
_____
_____

Recipe 182

CAROB ROMA COCONUT COOKIES

Place in a large bowl the following:

> One hundred almonds (roasted) cut in one half
> One teaspoon vanilla
> One cup maple syrup
> 4 teaspoons roma
> 4 tablespoons carob powder

Place in a vitamix or blender the following:

> 9 cups coconut (if blender cannot handle 9 cups at a time, then process 4 and half cups at a time)

Continue to blend until mixture is liquefied. Then pour into a large bowl with the above.

Mix,

On a cookie tray lined with parchment paper or a cookie mat, place the above mixture, One or Two spoons at a time on a sheet.

To form cookies, let cool and refrigerate.

Can freeze until needed

Notes: _____

_____

_____

Recipe 183

CAROB ICE CREAM

Place the following: in a vitamix or blender:

> One-fourth teaspoon
> Biosalt
> Two cups walnuts
> One brick or one pound tofu
> Three cups puffed rice
> Two cups maple syrup
> One tablespoon almond butter
> One half cup carob powder
> One half cup soymilk

Continue to blend until all ingredients are smooth

If too thick can add one tablespoon soymilk at a time

Freeze into 6 or 7 cups (6 ounce each cups)

Notes: _____

_____

_____

*Recipe 184*_____

CAROB CARMEL BARS

Place in a large bowl the following:

    One cup coconut
    One half cup carob powder
    One cup oatmeal flour
    One half cup maple syrup
    One half teaspoon Biosalt
    Two tablespoons almond butter
    One teaspoon rosewater

Mix and press into small dish, top with Two tablespoons chopped walnuts.

Refrigerate

Notes: _____
_____
_____

Recipe 185

CAROB SYRUP

Place in a vitamix or blender the following:

> One Cup hot water
> One and a half cups dates
> One Cup carob
> One fourth teaspoon rosewater
> One eighth teaspoon Biosalt

Blend until smooth

Can use as topping or a filling

Notes: _____

_____

_____

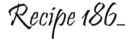

CAROB COCONUT FROSTING

In a vitamix or blender, place the following:

    Three fourths cup soymilk
    One half cup dates
    One half cup coconut
    Three fourths cup carob
    One fourth teaspoon Biosalt
    One half cup water
    One tablespoon rosewater

For cookies or cake, add one-half to one cup maple syrup

Notes: _____

_____

_____

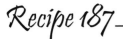 *Recipe 187*

SPECIAL SEASONING FOR ANYTHING

Place the following: in a vitamix or blender:

> One teaspoon parsley
> One teaspoon onion powder
> One teaspoon celery seeds or flakes
> One half teaspoon red pepper flakes
> One half teaspoon garlic powder
> One half teaspoon Marjoram
> One half teaspoon thyme
> One half teaspoon sage
> One half teaspoon savory
> One half teaspoon Biosalt

Then store in refrigerator

Notes: _____

_____

_____

*Recipe 188*_____

ITALIAN SALAD DRESSING

Place the following: in a vitamix or blender:

    One cup or 6 ounces cooked rice
    Three fourths cup water
    One teaspoon onion powder
    Two tablespoons Braggs amino
    One half cup or more lemon juice
    One teaspoon Italian seasoning
    One half teaspoon garlic powder
    One fourth teaspoon Biosalt

Then place in refrigerator

Notes: _____
_____
_____

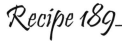*Recipe 189*

PINEAPPLE ICE CREAM

Place in a vitamix or blender the following:

    One half cup soymilk
    One Brick (or pound) tofu
    One fourth teaspoon Biosalt
    Two Cups maple syrup
    One tablespoon almond butter
    Two cups walnuts
    Three cups puffed rice
    One cup pineapple juice

Blend and freeze

Notes: _____
_____
_____

Recipe 190

ORANGE ICE CREAM

Place in a vitamix or blender the following:

    One half cup soymilk
    One Brick (or pound) tofu
    One fourth teaspoon Biosalt
    Two Cups maple syrup
    One tablespoon almond butter
    Two cups walnuts
    One cup orange juice or frozen juice
    Three cups puffed rice

Blend and freeze

Notes: _____

_____

_____

Recipe 191

CATSUP EXTRA

Place in a vitamix or blender the following:

Ingredients:

One and a half cups tomato paste
One and half cups water
One and half teaspoons onion powder
One fourth cup Lemon Juice
One half teaspoon Garlic Powder
One half teaspoon Biosalt
One half teaspoon Basil
One half teaspoon Paprika
One half teaspoon Dill Weed

Continue to blend.

Refrigerate or freeze the remainder

Notes: _____

_____

_____

Recipe 192———————————————————————

CHERRY ICE CREAM

Place in a vitamix or blender the following:

　　One half cup soymilk
　　One fourth teaspoon Biosalt
　　One cup cherries two cups walnuts
　　One brick or one pound tofu
　　Three cups puffed rice
　　Two cups maple syrup
　　One tablespoon almond butter

Blend, can place in six-ounce cups and freeze until ready to serve

Notes:　　　———————————————————————
　　　　　　———————————————————————
　　　　　　———————————————————————

Recipe 193

REAL COLORS FOR CAKES OR COOKIES

These colors to be used with whipped cream. (See recipe # 170)

This is not sweet; add any doughnut glaze under this topping.

Yellow - Use lemon cut off 90 % of color and remove all seeds

Red - Fresh cherries or red grapes

Orange - Remove orange color from outside can also use paprika or turmeric.

Peach - Use real dark colored peach with outside skin.

Green - Kiwi, remove brown skin, can keep seeds.

Purple - Use dark grapes or raspberries.

Place in vitamix or blender

Notes: _____

_____

_____

Recipe 194

CAROB PUDDING OR PIE FILLIING

Place in a vitamix or blender the following:

    One cup carob
    One fourth cup Tapioca
    Two tablespoons Roma
    One half teaspoon Biosalt
    One cup cooked rice
    Three fourths cup coconut
    Two tablespoons Rosewater
    One cup Maple Syrup
    Four packages (or four pounds) Tofu

Place in a dish and refrigerate. For pie place in a baked pie crust and refrigerate

Notes: _____

_____

_____

Recipe 195

ENGLISH TOFFEE COOKIES

Mix in a large bowl the following:

Ingredients:

One cup Almond Butter
One fourth cup Tofu
One teaspoon Cinnamon
One cup Sucanant Sugar
Two cups sifted Whole Wheat pastry flour

Mix and place into a cake pan 9x9 inch lined with parchment paper, with large spoon press dough into pan using back side large spoon. Add one cup chopped walnuts on top, and press into dough.

Bake at 275 degrees for one hour.

Let cool and cut into squares

Notes: _____

_____

_____

*Recipe 196*_____

CAROB CAKE FROSTING

Mix in a bowl the following:

One half cup almond butter
One fourth cup roma
One fourth cup carob

Place two and two thirds cup sucanant sugar into a vitamix to make into a powder, and then mix into the bowl with one teaspoon vanilla and 6 tablespoons soy milk. If too thick can add more soymilk; this will make Two cups

Notes: _____
_____
_____

Recipe 197

COCONUT CAKE

Place the following in a vitamix or blender:

    One Cup Almond Butter
    Two Cups Sucanant Sugar
    One Cup Coconut Flour
    One Cup Soymilk
    One-fourth teaspoonfuls Biosalt
    One Cup Tofu

Then pour into bowl and add 3 cups sifted whole-wheat pastry flour

Let sit until ingredients are at room temperature, then

Add one tablespoonful yeast, with ¼ cup finger warm water.

Mix and let sit for Two hours until dough rises

Mix and pour into cake pan or mold.

Bake at 350 degrees for 30 minutes or more.

Use the toothpick test in center, to see if the center is done

Let cool for One hour and add frosting. (See recipe No. 196)

Notes: _____

       _____

       _____

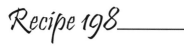

PUMPKIN COOKIES

In a large bowl, mix the following:

Ingredients:

Two cups Almond Butter
One cup Carob Powder
One cup Roma
Two cups Pumpkin (100%)
Two teaspoons Vanilla
One half cup Tofu
Two cups Maple syrup
Two cups sucanant Sugar
One half teaspoon Biosalt
Two teaspoons cinnamon
Two cups Oatmeal Flour
Four cups sifted Whole wheat Pastry Flour

Place mixture one to two spoons at a time on cookie sheets lined with parchment paper or a cookie mat. Form into shape.

Bake at 325 degrees for 30 minutes

Notes: _____

_____

_____

Recipe 199

BRAZIL NUT FUDGE

Boil for five minutes on warm, in a pan the following:

   Two and half cups sucanant sugar
   One cup maple sugar
   Stir and add one tablespoon roma powder
   One tablespoon carob powder

Boil for five minutes on warm:

Then add two cups Brazil nuts

Boil for five more minutes on warm

* cut each nut into four or five pieces, or smash nuts in a plastic bag with a rolling pin.

Stir and add two and half cups almond butter and boil on warm for five more minutes

Stir and pour into a 7 x 7 inch square glass dish lined with parchment paper

Cool and cut into squares

Notes: _____

_____

_____

Recipe 200

TAHEREH MALEK PUMPKIN ICE CREAM

Place the following: in a vitamix or blender:

Three cups puffed rice

One half cup soymilk

One pound or one brick tofu One fourth teaspoon Biosalt

One tablespoon almond butter

Two cups maple syrup

Two cups walnuts

Two cups pumpkin (if canned pumpkin being used

Ingredients should say 100% pumpkin only)

Continue to blend until smooth

Freeze in six-ounce cups

Notes: _____

_____

_____

Recipe 201

BAKED BROWN RICE

The night before place 4 cups rice and 7-8 cups water and one teaspoon Biosalt in a glass dish, with a lid: Stir

The next day mix and place into oven.

Bake for two hours at 250 degrees

After rice is cooked let sit to cool with lid on

Notes: _____

_____

_____

Recipe 202

GINGER CANDY

Boil on warm for 30 minutes the following:

6 cups Maple Syrup
3 Tablespoons Soymilk
One and one half teaspoonful Biosalt
6 Tablespoons Almond Butter

Add 3 Cups Puffed Rice and boil for 15 minutes on warm.

Add 4 teaspoons Ginger.

Boil for 15 more minutes on warm.

Add 3 cups Puffed Rice and boil for 15 minutes on low and stir until thick, and pour on two sheets parchment paper side by side, then place two more sheets on top and roll thin with a rolling pin.

Let cool and cut into squares

Notes: _____
_____
_____

Recipe 203

SANDRA MOONEY COFFEE CAKE

Place in a vitamix the following:

> One Brick or One pound Tofu, or Two cups Tofu
> 4 Teaspoonfuls if Vanilla
> Two Cups Soymilk
> Two Teaspoonfuls Biosalt

Mix and pour into a large bowl the following:

Six cups sifted whole-wheat pastry flour

Let sit until ingredients are room temperature

Then add Two tablespoons yeast

Mix with ¼-cup finger warm water

Let sit for two hours or until dough rises

Set aside.

Filling:

In a large bowl, mix the following:

> Eight tablespoonfuls almond butter
> One cup soymilk
> Two tablespoonfuls cinnamon
> Two tablespoonfuls Roma
> Four tablespoonfuls sifted whole-wheat pastry flour
> 8 cups or Two lbs Sucanant sugar/powder
> Six cups grounded walnuts

Next, this recipe makes Two cakes, two 9 x 9 lined pans with parchment paper needed

Mix and pour into pans, then pour batter

Bake 40 to 45 minutes at 350 degrees

Let cool and place in refrigerator for two hours or more

When cooled turn frosting side up

Notes: _____

_____

_____

Recipe 204

PAPAYA WALNUT COOKIES

Place the following in a vitamix:

    One Cup Almond Butter
    One Cup Maple Syrup
    One Cup Tofu
    One Cup Sucanant Sugar

Then pour into a large bowl with the following:

Two and a half cups sifted Whole wheat pastry flour

Two Cups Chopped Walnuts

Stir:

On Two-cookie trays line with parchment paper or a cookie mat, place and form

cookie dough into a ball like dome. Then press one piece dried papaya in center each cookie. Dried papaya should be size a dime.

Bake 20 minutes at 325 degrees

This recipe makes 24 cookies

Notes: _____

                 _____

                 _____

Recipe 205

LEMON CARROT COOKIES

Place the following in a vitamix:

> One-half teaspoonful Vanilla
> One Cup Almond Butter
> One Cup Maple syrup
> One and a half cups Sucanant sugar
> One half cup Lemon juice
> One fourth cup Tofu
> One-fourth teaspoonful Biosalt

Mix and pour into a large bowl with the following:

Two Cups sifted whole-wheat pastry flour

One and a half cups chopped walnuts

One` Cup shredded carrots

Place on Two trays using parchment paper or cookie mat.

This recipe makes 24 cookies.

Bake at 375 degrees for 12 minutes

Notes: _____

_____

_____

Recipe 206

CAROB SANDWICH COOKIES

Dough:

Place in a vitamix the following:

One and a half cups sucanant sugar
One cup Almond butter
One teaspoon vanilla
One fourth cup tofu
One half teaspoon Biosalt
One fourth cup soymilk

Mix, and pour into a large bowl and add:

One third cup Carob
One and a half cups sifted whole wheat pastry flour

Mix and place in a pan 11 X 9 inch square, lined pan with parchment paper.

Bake 11 -12 minutes at 350 degrees.

Use toothpick test to see if center is done. Let cool and place in refrigerator.

Filling:

In a bowl, mix the following:

Two cups sucanant sugar
One half teaspoon vanilla
One fourth cup Almond butter and two tablespoons Almond butter

Add soymilk, one teaspoon at a time until filling is smooth and creamy.

Then mix and set aside.

After dough has been cooled cut dough- cake in half. Remove from parchment paper, and then place a thin layer filling on each side. Then place on top each other, like a sandwich. Then return to refrigerator for at least One hour or more.

Before serving cut into small squares

Notes: _____

_____

_____

Recipe 207

DAISY FROSTING

Mix in a bowl the following:

Ingredients:

> Two tablespoons Almond Butter
> Three tablespoons Soy Milk
> One half cup Sucanant Sugar
> One and one half cups Chopped Walnuts

Mix and spread while cake is still hot.

Can put cake back in oven, until frosting is bubbly, then let cool and refrigerate

Notes: _____

_____

_____

Recipe 208

BLACK EYED PEAS

The night before soak one pound Black Eyed Peas in enough water 3 to 4 inches above the peas.

The next day boil 10 minutes and change the water, and add:

One completely raw potato
One Tablespoonful Biosalt
One Onion chopped
One half cup Cilantro
One Teaspoonful Garlic Powder
One Tablespoonful Braggs Ammino

Add enough water to boil peas approximately 30 - 40 minutes in pan.

After peas are cooked, throw potato away.

Can freeze extra

Notes: _____

_____

_____

Recipe 209

ALMOND BUTTER FROSTING

Place the following in a vitamix:

8 Cups Sucanant Sugar -- make into a fine powder.

Then pour into a bowl with the following:

> One half cup Soymilk
> Two teaspoonfuls Vanilla
> One-half teaspoonful Biosalt
> One cup Almond Butter

Mix

If mixture is too thick, add more soymilk, and then apply at room temperature to cake or cookies.

Then refrigerate

Notes: _____

_____

_____

*Recipe 210*_____

TOFU FROSTING

Place in a vitamix or blender the following:

    Two teaspoons vanilla
    Two cups sucanant sugar
    One fourth cup tofu and one half cup tofu
    One half cup almond butter

Mix and apply at room temperature to cake and cookies, then refrigerate

Notes: _____
                    _____
                    _____

Recipe 211

CHERI GILBERT
COOKED CAROB GLAZE

In a pan, boil the following:

> One Tablespoonful Almond Butter
> One Tablespoonful Roma
> One Tablespoonful Carob
> Two Tablespoonfuls water or soymilk
> Two thirds cup Sucanant Sugar
> One-fourth teaspoonful Vanilla

Continue to boil on warm and stir until thick. If too thick can add extra soymilk

Cool at room temperature and apply to cake or cookies.

Then refrigerate

Notes: _____

_____

_____

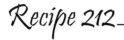Recipe 212

SUCANANT SUGAR GLAZE

Place the following in a vitamix:

    One Tablespoonful Lemon Juice
    6 to 8 Tablespoonfuls Hot Soy Milk
    Two and half cups Sucanant Sugar

Mix and cool.

Apply at room temperature to top of cake or cookies and refrigerate

Notes: _____

_____

_____

Recipe 213

ROMA CREAM FROSTING

Place in a bowl the following:

One and a half cups almond butter
One teaspoon vanilla
One and a half cups sucanant sugar
Two tablespoons carob
Three tablespoons roma
One eighth teaspoon Biosalt
Three tablespoons soymilk

Mix and add to cooled baked cakes or cookies

Apply at room temperature

Cool and refrigerate

Notes: _____

_____

_____

Recipe 214

LEMON FILLING

Place the following: in a vitamix or blender:

> One half cup sucanant sugar
> Two tablespoons whole-wheat pastry flour
> Two thirds cup water or soymilk
> One eighth teaspoon Biosalt
> 3 tablespoons lemon juice
> One half teaspoon grated lemon juice

Mix until thick then add one half cup tofu and one fourth cup tofu..., and then two tablespoons almond butter.

Mix until thick and add to pie or pastry

Notes: _____
_____
_____

Recipe 215

BAR - B -QUE SAUCE

Place in a small pan the following:

>   One cup hot sauce
>   One third cup Braggs Ammino
>   One teaspoon chili powder
>   One teaspoon Biosalt
>   Two cups water

Bring to a boil, then turn to low for approximately 15 minutes, let cool and freeze until needed

Notes: _____

_____

_____

Recipe 216

TOFU FROSTING

Place in a vitamix all the following:

  Two Teaspoons Vanilla
  Two Cups Sucanat sugar
  One fourth cup Tofu and one half cup Tofu
  One half cup almond butter

If too thick can add soymilk one teaspoonful at a time

Mix and apply at room temperature to cake or cookies. Then refrigerate

Notes: _____

_____

_____

Recipe 217

SWEET SUGAR ICING

Place into a vitamix the following:

One cup sucanant sugar
Then pour into a bowl with the following:
One teaspoon vanilla
One teaspoon soy milk

Stir and if mixture is too thick can add more soy milk, one teaspoon at a time.

Apply at room temperature to cake or cookies and refrigerate

Notes: _____

_____

_____

*Recipe 218*_____

BLACK EYED PEAS IN RICE

Boil the following in a pan:

> One half teaspoon marjoram
> One tablespoons Braggs Ammino
> One half cup cilantro (chopped)
> One teaspoon Biosalt
> One onion chopped
> One tablespoon chili powder
> One bell pepper cut small

Boil for 15 minutes and let sit, and then add 12 ounces cooked Black Eyed Peas and stir. Add to cooked rice and stir and let sit with lid on rice pan, with stove off. (Rice should be cooked at the same time as the above)

Notes: _____

_____

_____

Recipe 219

SOY MILK CORNBREAD

Place in a vitamix the following:

Two teaspoons sucanant sugar
8 Teaspoons Almond butter
One half cup tofu
4 teaspoons Biosalt
Three cups soymilk

Mix, and place into a large bowl with the following:

Two cups whole corn
Two cups corn meal
Two cups sifted whole-wheat pastry flour

Let sit until all ingredients are at room temperature then

Add

One tablespoonful yeast in ¼ cup finger temperature water

Let sit for Two hours or until dough rises

Mix and add to a pan 11 X 9 inch glass dish lined pan with parchment paper.

If you want thicker bread, use a smaller dish.

Bake 20 minutes at 425 degrees

Notes: _____

_____

_____

Recipe 220

OATMEAL ALMOND COOKIES

Place in a bowl the following:

> 6 cups Oatmeal flour
> Two Cups sucanant sugar/flour
> Two cups sifted whole-wheat pastry flour
> One half teaspoon Clove powder
> One teaspoon Biosalt
> Two teaspoons cinnamon

Place the following in a vitamix:

> One cup tofu
> Two cups Maple syrup
> Two Cups Almond Butter
> Two Teaspoons o f Vanilla

Mix and add to above bowl. Stir and form cookies on tray lined with parchment paper or a cookie mat.

Bake at 350 degrees for 15 minutes

Notes: _____
_____
_____

Recipe 221

SPICE CUP CAKES

Place in a vitamix the following:

> Two cups sucanant sugar flour
> Two cups soymilk
> Two teaspoons cinnamon
> One teaspoon ground cloves
> One half teaspoon Biosalt
> One cup tofu

Mix, then pour into a bowl with the following:

Three cups sifted whole-wheat pastry flour

Let sit until all ingredients are at room temperature then

Add

> One tablespoonful yeast in ¼ cup finger temperature water
> Let sit for two hours or until dough rises
> Stir and place into cup cake holders, then place in muffin pans.

Bake 15 minutes at 375 degrees.

Use toothpick test to see if baked.

Place frosting while still warm. Then place in refrigerator, can freeze extra.

This recipe makes 26-cup cakes

Notes: _____

_____

_____

Recipe 222

DATE OATMEAL COOKIES

PLACE IN A VITAMIX THE FOLLOWING:

Two cups sucanant sugar
Two cups almond butter
One cup tofu
Two teaspoons vanilla
Two teaspoons cinnamon
One teaspoon Biosalt

Mix and pour into a bowl with the following:

Two cups pecans (grinded)
Three cups dates (chopped)
Four cups oatmeal flour
Three and a half cups sifted whole wheat pastry
flour

Mix and pour into a cake pan - the size depends on how thick you want your cookie to be.

Bake 375 degrees for 10 to 12 minutes or until baked. Let cool completely, and refrigerate for approximately 2 hours. Cut into wedges or desired shapes

Notes: _____

_____

_____

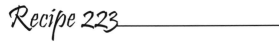

ORANGE COCONUT COOKIES

Place in a vitamix the following:

    Two cups Maple syrup
    Two Cups Almond Butter
    Two Teaspoons o f Vanilla
    One half Cup Tofu
    One half Teaspoon Biosalt
    Five teaspoons grated orange peel

Mix and pour into a bowl with following:

Two and a half Cups Dry Coconut

Five Cups sifted whole-wheat pastry flour

Mix to form cookies.

Place on cookie tray lined with parchment paper or a cookie mat.

Bake at 375 degrees for 13 to 15 minutes

Notes: _____

_____

_____

Recipe 224

DATE BAR COOKIES

Dough:

Place in a vitamix the following:

    One cup Maple syrup
    One cup tofu
    One cup Sucanant sugar
    One cup Almond butter
    One teaspoon vanilla
    One half teaspoon Biosalt

Mix, and add to a bowl with:

One half cup wheat germ

Two and half cups sifted whole-wheat pastry flour

Mix and let set for Two hours.

Using a rolling pins - roll out dough thin, a shape 12 x 16 inches. This is size of a cookie mat.

Use extra whole-wheat pastry flour - dough should not stick to cookie mat. Cut rectangular lengthwise into thirds. Spread dried fruit down the center of each strip. Fold sides over filling to overlap. Cut into one and half-inch bars and place on cookie trays lined with parchment paper or a cookie mat. Cut with a plastic knife.

Bake 20 minutes at 375 degrees.

Filling:

Place in a vitamix the following:

    6 tablespoons Lemon juice
    6 cups dates

Two cups Sucanant sugar
One cup hot water

Mix and pour into a bowl with:

One cup grinded walnuts

Notes: _____

_____

_____

Recipe 225

APRICOT BAR COOKIES

DOUGH:

Place in a vitamix the following:

    One cup maple syrup
    One cup tofu
    One cup sucanant sugar
    One cup almond butter
    One teaspoon vanilla
    One half teaspoon Biosalt

Mix and add to a bowl with:

    One half cup wheat germ
    Two and half cups sifted whole-wheat pastry flour

Mix and let set for Two hours

FILLING:

Place in a small pan the following:

    One cup chopped walnuts
    Two cup sucanant sugar
    One cup water
    Two tablespoons grated orange peel
    6 cups dried apricots, cut small

Heat on medium for 5 - 8 minutes or until thick

Let cool completely, Mixture will be thick

Notes: _____

_____

_____

Recipe 226

GINGER BREAD PANCAKES

Place in a vitamix the following:

> One fourth teaspoon Biosalt
> One teaspoon cinnamon
> Three fourths cup soymilk
> One fourth teaspoon clove powder
> One half cup tofu
> One fourth teaspoon maple syrup
> 3 teaspoons almond butter
> One teaspoons ginger
> One and a half cups sifted whole-wheat pastry flour

For cooking - follow pancake instructions or heat a large non-stick pan over medium heat, then drop batter one cup at a time. When small bubbles appear, flip the pancake over and continue to cook approximately 3 to 4 minutes total. (Both sides)

Can freeze extra

Notes: _____

_____

_____

Recipe 227

LEMON PASTRY

Place in a large bowl the following:

Two cups Almond butter
Two cups Maple syrup
Two cups walnuts chopped
Two cups sifted whole-wheat pastry flour

Mix and Place on cookie tray lined with parchment paper.

Bake 350 degrees for 25 minutes.

For topping:

Place the following in a vitamix:

6 tablespoons lemon juice
Two cups maple syrup
One cup Sucanant sugar
One brick tofu
One third cup whole-wheat pastry flour
6 tablespoons grated lemon rind, or to taste

Mix and add topping to baked crust. Then add to top Two cups of chopped walnuts.

Return to oven for 25 - 30 minutes at 350 degrees

Notes: _____

_____

_____

Recipe 228

LEMON SUGARCOOKIES

Place in a vitamix the following:

> 2 Cups Almond Butter
> Two Teaspoons o f Vanilla
> Two Teaspoons grated Lemon peel
> One half cup tofu
> Two Cups Maple syrup
> Two Cups Sucanant sugar

Mix and pour into a large bowl with following:

One teaspoon Biosalt

Then add 4 cups sifted whole-wheat pastry flour.

Stir all the above, using three cookie trays lined with parchment paper or a cookie mat.

Form cookies on tray.

Bake at 375 degrees for 15 minutes

Notes: _____
_____
_____

Recipe 229

DATE BROWNIES

Place in a vitamix the following:

One Cup Almond Butter
2 Teaspoons o f Vanilla
One cup tofu
Two Cups Maple syrup
One Teaspoon Biosalt
One and half cups Carob

Mix and pour into a large bowl with following:

Two Cups chopped walnuts
Two Cups chopped dates (cut each into 5 to 6 parts)
Two Cups sifted whole-wheat pastry flour
When all ingredients are room temperature

Add

One tablespoonful yeast in ¼ cup finger temperature water

Let sit for two hours or until dough rises

Mix and pour into a 9 x 13 inch glass dish lined with parchment paper.

Bake at 350 degrees for 35 - 45 minutes.

Use toothpick test to see if center is done

When cool cut into squares

Notes: _____
_____
_____

*Recipe 230*_____

ORIGINAL SALT WATER TAFFY

In a small pan, boil the following on warm for 30 minutes:

    One Cup Sucanant sugar
    Two Tablespoonfuls Corn starch
    One-half teaspoonful Biosalt
    One Cup Maple syrup
    One half cup Water
    Two Tablespoonfuls Almond Butter
    Before turning off heat, see the freezer test

Continue to boil and stir.

Turn off heat. Let cool in pan for 10 minutes. Then pour two teaspoonfuls vanilla on top - do not stir - with a plastic knife spread vanilla. Then pour mixture on top of cookie mat and let cool.

Cut or break into squares and wrap each in wax paper.

Note: Heat from stoves can vary. Too much heat will make taffy hard and not enough heat will make taffy too soft. If too soft can place in refrigerator If too hard make correction next time. (Heat and stirring will make the biggest recipe difference)

Freezer test: place a few drops of the mixture on the cookie mat and place into freezer for 30 seconds

If mixture is soft/repeat freezer test

If mixture is harder, turn off stovetop

Notes: _____

                 _____

                 _____

Recipe 231 ————————————————

AURA VICTORIA HUCK PEPPERMINT SALT WATER TAFFY

In a small pan, boil the following on WARM for 30 minutes:

    One Cup sucanant sugar
    Two tablespoons cornstarch
    One half cup mint water
    One cup maple syrup
    One half teaspoon Biosalt
    Two tablespoons almond butter
    1/4 teaspoon peppermint oil
    See freezer test

Continue to stir and boil.

Turn off heat.

Let cool for 10 minutes

Then pour Two teaspoons vanilla on top -- do not stir -- with a plastic knife spread vanilla. Then pour mixture on top of cookie mat and let cool. Cut or break into one-inch squares and wrap each in wax paper.

Note: Heat from stoves can vary, too much heat will make taffy hard and not enough heat will make taffy too soft, if too soft can place in refrigerator. If too hard, make correction next time.

(Heat and stirring will make the biggest recipe difference)

Freezer test: place a few drops of the mixture on the cookie mat and place into freezer for 30 seconds

If mixture is soft/repeat freezer test

If mixture is harder, turn off stovetop

Notes:

_____

_____

_____

Recipe 232

LEMON SALT WATER TAFFY

In a small pan, boil the following on warm for 30 minutes:

> One Cup Sucanant sugar
> Two Tablespoonfuls Corn starch
> One-half teaspoon Biosalt
> One Cup Maple syrup
> One half cup Lemon juice
> Two Tablespoons Almond Butter
> Two to 5 Tablespoons Lemon Rind, or to taste
> Before turning off heat, see the freezer test

Continue to boil and stir.

Turn off heat. Let cool in pan for 10 minutes. Then pour two teaspoonfuls vanilla on top - do not stir - with a plastic knife spread vanilla. Then pour mixture on top of cookie mat and let cool.

Cut or break into squares and wrap each in wax paper.

Note: Heat from stoves can vary. Too much heat will make taffy hard and not enough heat will make taffy too soft. If too soft can place in refrigerator, if too hard make correction next time (Heat and stirring will make the biggest recipe difference)

Freezer test: place a few drops of the mixture on the cookie mat and place into freezer for 30 seconds

If mixture is soft/repeat freezer test

If mixture is harder, turn off stovetop

Frederick Mickel Huck

Notes:

_____

_____

_____

Recipe 233

VANILLA SALT WATER TAFFY

In a small pan, boil the following on WARM for 30 minutes:

> One Cup sucanant sugar
> Two tablespoons cornstarch
> One half cup water
> Two teaspoons vanilla or to your taste
> One cup maple syrup
> One half teaspoon Biosalt
> Two tablespoons almond butter
> See freezer test

Continue to stir and boil.

Turn off heat.

Let cool for 10 minutes

Then pour Two teaspoons vanilla on top -- do not stir -- with a plastic knife spread vanilla. Then pour mixture on top of cookie mat and let cool. Cut or break into one-inch squares and wrap each in wax paper.

Note: Heat from stoves can vary, too much heat will make taffy hard and not enough heat will make taffy too soft, if too soft can place in refrigerator. If too hard, make correction next time.

(Heat and stirring will make the biggest recipe difference)

Freezer test: place a few drops of the mixture on the cookie mat and place into freezer for 30 seconds

If mixture is soft/repeat freezer test

If mixture is harder, turn off stovetop

Notes:
_____

_____

_____

Recipe 234

ORANGE SALT WATER TAFFY

In a small pan, boil the following on warm for 30 minutes:

One Cup Sucanant sugar

Two Tablespoonfuls Corn starch

One-half teaspoonful Biosalt

One Cup Maple syrup

One half cup Orange juice

Two Tablespoonfuls Almond Butter

3 Tablespoonfuls Orange Rind or to taste

Before turning off heat, see freezer test

Continue to boil and stir.

Turn off heat. Let cool in pan for 10 minutes. Then pour two teaspoonfuls vanilla on top - do not stir - with a plastic knife spread vanilla. Then pour mixture on top of cookie mat and let cool.

Cut or break into squares and wrap each in wax paper.

Note: Heat from stoves can vary. Too much heat will make taffy hard and not enough heat will make taffy too soft. If taffy is too soft, place in the refrigerator until firm. If too hard, make correction next time. (Heat and stirring will make the biggest recipe difference)

Freezer test: place a few drops of the mixture on the cookie mat and place into freezer for 30 seconds

If mixture is soft/repeat freezer test

If mixture is harder, turn off stovetop

Notes:

_____

_____

_____

Recipe 235

JACK PANAGOPOULOS ROMA SALT WATER TAFFY

In a small pan, boil the following on warm for 30 minutes:

One Cup sucanant sugar

Two tablespoons cornstarch

One half cup water

One cup maple syrup

One half teaspoon Biosalt

Two tablespoons roma

Two tablespoons almond butter

See freezer test

Continue to stir and boil.

Turn off heat.

Let cool in pan for 10 minutes,

Then pour Two teaspoons vanilla on top -- do not stir -- with a plastic knife spread vanilla. Then pour mixture on top of cookie mat and let cool. Cut or break into one-inch squares and wrap each in wax paper.

Note: Heat from stoves can vary, too much heat will make taffy hard and not enough heat will make taffy too soft, if too soft can place in refrigerator. If too hard, make correction next time.

(Heat and stirring will make the biggest recipe difference)

Freezer test: place a few drops of the mixture on the cookie mat and place into freezer for 30 seconds

If mixture is soft/repeat freezer test

If mixture is harder, turn off stovetop

Notes: _____

_____

_____

Recipe 236

ADRIANA CERRILL0 PECAN SALT WATER TAFFY

In a small pan, boil the following on warm for 30 minutes:

> One Cup Sucanant sugar
> Two Tablespoons Corn starch
> One half cup water
> One Cup Maple syrup
> Two Tablespoons Almond butter
> One half teaspoon Biosalt
> One Cup grounded Pecans
> See freezer test

Continue to boil and stir.

Turn off heat.

Let cool in pan for 10 minutes.

The pour Two teaspoons vanilla on top - do not stir - with a plastic knife spread vanilla then pour mixture on top of cookie mat and let cool.

Cut or break into squares and wrap each in wax paper.

Note: Heat from stoves can vary, too much heat will make taffy hard and not enough heat will make taffy too soft. If too soft can place in refrigerator. If too hard, make correction next time.

(Heat and stirring will make the biggest recipe difference)

Freezer test: place a few drops the mixture on the cookie mat and place into freezer for 30 seconds

If mixture is soft/repeat freezer test

If mixture is harder, turn off stovetop

Notes:
_____
_____
_____

Recipe 237

ALMOND SALT WATER TAFFY

In a small pan, boil the following on medium for 20 minutes:

    One Cup sucanant sugar
    Two tablespoons cornstarch
    One half cup water
    One cup maple syrup
    One half teaspoon Biosalt
    Two tablespoons almond butter
    One cup grounded almonds

Continue to stir and boil.

Turn off heat.

Let cool in pan for 10 minutes,

Then pour Two teaspoons vanilla on top -- do not stir -- with a plastic knife spread vanilla. Then pour mixture on top of cookie mat and let cool. Cut or break into one inch squares and wrap each in wax paper.

Note: Heat from stoves can vary, too much heat will make taffy hard and not enough heat will make taffy too soft, if too soft can place in refrigerator. If too hard, make correction next time.

(Heat and stirring will make the biggest recipe difference)

Notes: _____

        _____

        _____

Recipe 238

ASHELY SPEIDELL WALNUT SALT WATER TAFFY

In a small pan, boil the following on warm for 30 minutes:

   One Cup sucanant sugar
   Two tablespoons cornstarch
   One half cup water
   One cup maple syrup
   One half teaspoon Biosalt
   Two tablespoons almond butter
   One cup walnuts chopped
   See freezer test

Continue to stir and boil.

Turn off heat.

Let cool in pan for 10 minutes,

Then pour Two teaspoons vanilla on top -- do not stir -- with a plastic knife spread vanilla. Then pour mixture on top of cookie mat and let cool. Cut or break into one inch squares and wrap each in wax paper.

Note: Heat from stoves can vary, too much heat will make taffy hard and not enough heat will make taffy too soft, if too soft can place in refrigerator. If too hard, make correction next time.

(Heat and stirring will make the biggest recipe difference)

Freezer test: place a few drops of the mixture on the cookie mat and place into freezer for 30 seconds

If mixture is soft/repeat freezer test

If mixture is harder, turn off stovetop

Notes:

_____

_____

_____

Recipe 239————————————————————————

ROSS H. MENZIE CAROB SALT WATER TAFFY

In a small pan, boil the following on warm for 30 minutes:

    One Cup Sucanant sugar
    Two Tablespoonfuls Corn starch
    One half teaspoonfuls Biosalt
    One Cup Maple syrup
    One half cup water
    Two Tablespoonfuls Almond Butter
    Two Tablespoonfuls Carob
    Before turning off heat, see freezer test

Continue to boil and stir.

Turn off heat. Let cool in pan for 10 minutes. Then pour two teaspoonfuls vanilla on top - do not stir - with a plastic knife spread vanilla. Then pour mixture on top of cookie mat and let cool.

Cut or break into squares and wrap each in wax paper.

Note: Heat from stoves can vary. Too much heat will make taffy hard and not enough heat will make taffy too soft. If too soft can place in refrigerator. If too hard, make correction next time. (Heat and stirring will make the biggest recipe difference)

Freezer test: place a few drops of the mixture on the cookie mat and place into freezer for 30 seconds

If mixture is soft/repeat freezer test

If mixture is harder, turn off stovetop

Notes: _____

_____

_____

Recipe 240

COCONUT SALT WATER TAFFY

In a small pan, boil the following on warm for 30 minutes:

One Cup Sucanant sugar
Two Tablespoons Corn starch
One half teaspoon Biosalt
Two Tablespoons Coconut flour
One Cup Maple syrup
One half cup Coconut milk or water
Two Tablespoons Almond butter
See freezer test

Continue to boil and stir.

Turn off heat.

Let cool in pan for 10 minutes.

Then pour Two teaspoons vanilla on top - do not stir - with a plastic knife spread vanilla , then pour mixture on top of cookie mat and let cool.

Cut or break into squares and wrap each in wax paper.

Note: Heat from stoves can vary, too much heat will make taffy hard and not enough heat will make taffy too soft. If too soft can place in refrigerator. If too hard, make correction next time.

(Heat and stirring will make the biggest recipe difference)

Freezer test: place a few drops of the mixture on the cookie mat and place into freezer for 30 seconds

If mixture is soft/repeat freezer test

If mixture is harder, turn off stovetop

Notes:

_____

_____

_____

Recipe 241

CINNAMON SALT WATER TAFFY

In a small pan, boil the following on warm for 30 minutes:

> One Cup Sucanant sugar
> Two Tablespoons Corn starch
> One half teaspoon Biosalt
> One-Two Tablespoons Cinnamon
> One Cup Maple syrup
> One half cup water
> Two Tablespoons Almond butter
> See freezer test

Continue to boil and stir.

Turn off heat.

Let cool in pan for 10 minutes.

Then pour Two teaspoons vanilla on top - do not stir - with a plastic knife spread vanilla then pour mixture on top of cookie mat and let cool.

Cut or break into squares and wrap each in wax paper.

Note: Heat from stoves can vary, too much heat will make taffy hard and not enough heat will make taffy too soft. If too soft can place in refrigerator. If too hard, make correction next time.
(Heat and stirring will make the biggest recipe difference)

Freezer test: place a few drops the mixture on the cookie mat and place into freezer for 30 seconds

If mixture is soft/repeat freezer test

If mixture is harder, turn off stovetop

Notes:

_____

_____

_____

Recipe 242

GINGER SALT WATER TAFFY

In a small pan, boil the following on warm for 30 minutes:

> One Cup Sucanant sugar
> Two Tablespoonfuls Corn starch
> One half teaspoonfuls Biosalt
> One Teaspoonful Ginger
> One Cup Maple syrup
> One half cup water
> Two Tablespoonfuls Almond Butter
> Before turning off heat, see freezer test

Continue to boil and stir.

Turn off heat. Let cool in pan for 10 minutes. Then pour two teaspoonfuls vanilla on top - do not stir - with a plastic knife spread vanilla. Then pour mixture on top of cookie mat and let cool.

Cut or break into squares and wrap each in wax paper.

Note: Heat from stoves can vary. Too much heat will make taffy hard and not enough heat will make taffy too soft. If too soft can place in refrigerator. If too hard, make correction next time. (Heat and stirring will make the biggest recipe difference)

Freezer test: place a few drops of the mixture on the cookie mat and place into freezer for 30 seconds

If mixture is soft/repeat freezer test

If mixture is harder, turn off stove top

Notes: _____

_____

_____

Recipe 243

GENE KOENIG ENGLISH TOFFEE CANDY

In a large pan, boil for 30 minutes on warm the following:

    3 tablespoons soymilk
    One and half teaspoons Biosalt
    6 tablespoons almond butter
    6 cups maple syrup

Continue to boil and stir. Add one cup roma, and continue to boil on warm for 15 more minutes.

Add 3 cups roasted grounded almonds, and continue to boil for 15 more minutes.

Add 3 cups puffed rice and continue to boil on warm 15 more minutes. Continue to boil and stir until thick or like oatmeal.

Can turn heat low - must stir continuously.

When mixture is thick pour on parchment paper, four sheets needed, use two on the bottom, and then two sheets on top with a rolling pin press thin

Let cool. Refrigerate extra

Notes: _____

_____

_____

Recipe 244

LUCILLE GILBERT LEMON CHEESE CAKE

Crust:

Make crust first, see special piecrust recipe # 38 -- Do not add any maple syrup.

Mix and add crust into 10 X 3 inch spring form pan lined with parchment paper.

Filling:

Place the following into a vitamix.

> Two cups tofu
> One cup soymilk
> Two tablespoons lemon juice
> One teaspoon vanilla
> One and a half cups sucanant sugar
> One fourth cup whole-wheat pastry flour

Mix and pour into a pan.

Bake One hour and 15 minutes at 325 degrees

Notes: _____
_____
_____

Recipe 245

ORANGE CHEESE CAKE

Crust:

Make crust first

See special piecrust
Recipe #38 - do not add any maple syrup.

Mix and add crust into 10 x 10:

 Three inch or deeper spring form pan
 lined with parchment paper.

Filling:

Place the following into a vitamix:

 Two cups tofu
 One cup soy milk
 Two teaspoons orange rind
 Two tablespoons orange juice
 One tablespoon vanilla
 One and a half cups sucanant sugar
 One fourth cup whole wheat pastry flour

Mix and pour into a pan.

Bake one hour and fifteen minutes at 325 degrees

Notes: _____

_____

_____

_____

Recipe List

1. BAKED POTATO
2. SALADS
3. PASTA
4. PASTA SAUCE - TOMATO SAUCE
5. BROWN RICE
6. TEXAN RICE
7   BELL PEPPER RICE
8. TOSTADAS
9. POPCORN
10. HOT SAUCE
11. CINDY HUCK BEANS FOR BURRITOS
12. TODD NEUMILLER CHINESE SOUP
13. ALMOND BUTTER
14. PIZZA SAUCE
15. PIZZA DOUGH (FOR PIES)
16. WAFFLES
17. TAMALE CASSEROLE
18. MAPLE SYRUP CAKE
19. PAN - FRIED NOODLES
20. FRUIT ICING
21. CAROB BAKED ALASKA
22. VANILLA CAKE
23. CAROB GLAZE
24. MAPLE OATMEAL CAKE
25. CLOVE COOKIES
26. DONALD W. HUCK COCONUT COOKIES

27. CAROB ROMA OATMEAL COOKIES

28. DEEP - DISH PIZZA

29. COCONUT OATMEAL CAROB ROMA COOKIES

30. COCONUT OATMEAL COOKIES

31. CAROB ROMA COCONUT OATMEAL WHOLE-WHEAT PASTRY FLOUR COOKIES

32. COCONUT OATMEAL WHOLE WHEAT PASTRY FLOUR COOKIES

33. STUFFED BELL PAPPERS

34. MAPLE SYRUP COOKIES

35. CAROB COOKIES

36. CAROB BROWN CAKE

37. ANY FRUIT COOKIES (PEACH, CHERRY, APRICOT)

38. SPECIAL PIE CRUST

39. PUMPKIN PIE

40. PARVIN MALEK CAROB PIE

41. ALMOND BUTTER COOKIES 2

42. CAROB FILLING

43. EVELYN ANN MENZIE OLD-FASHIONED GLAZE

44. PINEAPPLE PIE

45. BUTTER COOKIES

46. SUCANANT COOKIES

47. INEZ A.   MENZIE COCONUT COOKIES

48. TURNOVERS

49. GOLDEN MACAROONS

50. ORIENTAL CRUNCH

51. PINEAPPLE CANDY

52. CAROB DOUGHNUTS

53. LEMON DOUGHNUTS

54. GRAIN PIZZA

55. CORNMEAL PIZZA

56. CAROB BROWNIES

57. ROBERT E MENZIE WALNUT PIE

58. APRICOT COCONUT WALNUT SQUARES

59. PISTACHIO SCONES

60. EGG ROLLS

61. ROASTED SALTED NUTS

62. FUDGE CUP COOKIE

63. FUDGE SAUCE

64. PINEAPPLE COOKIES

65. TAMALE BEAN PIE

66. NUT PIE

67. DATE WALNUT COOKIES

68. CARAMELIZED GINGER HAZELNUT TART

69. PAPAYA COOKIES

70. CAJUN MIXED NUTS

71. TACO SALAD SHELLS

72. FOR CAKE-WEDDING STYLE CAKE

73. SPANISH MILLET CASSEROLE

74. ENCHILADAS

75. CAROB PIE

76. NUT BUTTER BALLS

77. SHARAREH SHABAFROOZ GARLIC BREAD SPREAD/BUTTER

78. GLAZED CARROT CAKE

79. WAFFLES WITH CASHEWS AND OATMEAL

80. LEMON PINEAPPLE PIE

81. CORN BREAD

82. MATTHEW F. MOONEY ROAST FOR ANY HOLIDAY

83. SPICE DOUGHNUTS

84. SPANISH RICE

85. PINEAPPLE SANDWICH COOKIE

86. CAROB CUP COOKIE

87. ANY FRUIT CUP COOKIE

88. SETAREH TAIS CAKE

89. CAROB DATE PISTACHIO PASTRY

90. FRUIT CAKE COOKIE

91. BAKED MILLET

92. BISCOTTI

93. MULTIGRAIN CRACKERS

94. POT PIE

95. BASIC COOKIE WITH FROSTING

96. TACO SHELLS

97. ANY FRUIT PASTRY

98. PINEAPPLE FROSTING

99. PINEAPPLE UPSIDE DOWN CAKE

100. HOT BEANS FOR BURRITOS

101. APRICOT PIE

102. APPLE PIE

103. PLUM PIE

104. PIZZA SAUCE NO. 3

105. PIZZA SAUCE NO. 1

106. COFFEE MUFFINS

107. GLORIA DUGGINS PECAN CANDY

108. PETER P.   PANAGOPOULOS ALMOND FUDGE

109. PETE/ROSA CERRILLO CINNAMON WALNUT CANDY

110. SUGARED NUTS

111. PAPAYA CANDY

112. CAROB CAKE

113. THELMA MAIN HAZELNUT FUDGE

114. WHEAT CORNMEAL PIZZA

115. MARGARET/HARVEY BINDER PECAN FUDGE

116. MICHAEL F. MOONEY PECAN ROMA CAROB CANDY

117. BELLE HUCK WALNUT FUDGE

118. SAUCE FOR INSIDE CINNAMON ROLLS

119. NECTARINE PIE

120. COOKIES/CAROB PLAIN OR ROMA

121. CAROB BARS

122. SPICE BUTTER COOKIES

123. OAT CRACKERS

124. CINNAMON SUGAR DOUGHNUT TOPPING

125. JELLY DOUGHNUT FILLING

126. STRUDEL DOUGH

127. DATE CUP COOKIE

128. ITALIAN SAUCE

129. LASAGNA

130. BOB PANAGOPOULOS PIZZA SAUCE NO. 2

131. CUBAN BLACK BEANS IN RICE

132. BLACK BEANS

133. LIGHT FUDGE

134. DARK FUDGE

135. PIGEON BEANS

136. XENIA PANAGOPOULOS PIGEON RICE

137. ALEXANDRA PANAGOPOULOS SWEET AND SOUR SAUCE NO. 1

138. INEZ SPEIDELL SWEET AND SOUR SAUCE NO. 2

139. VERY VERY HOT SAUCE

140. LENTILS

141. SHRIMP SAUCE

142. GABRIEL CERRILLO ALMOND CAROB CANDY

143. CAROB ROMA CANDY

144. WALNUT CINNAMON CLUSTERS

145. TAMARA NEUMILLER SPANISH PASTA

146. CHINESE RICE

147. CHILI BEANS

148. TAMALES

149. VEGETABLE SOUP

150. CAROB ROMA COOKIES

151. RAY AND LINDA PANAGOPOULOS SUNFLOWER COCONUT WAFFLES

152. WAFFLES OATMEAL AND ALMONDS

153. RHI CAROB AND ROMA OATMEAL WWP NUTLESS COOKIE

154. HOT SAUCE

155. RED BEANS FOR TOP OF RICE

156. CORN MEAL WAFFLES

157. TAGLIATELLE SAUCE

158. ALMOND BUTTER COOKIES

159. MAPLE SYRUP FROSTING

160. ORANGE GLAZE

161. RYE PANCAKES

162. PANCAKES

163. BLUEBERRY TOPPING

164. ROMA ICE CREAM

165. LEMON ICE CREAM

166. ORANGE DATE SYRUP

167. CAROB FUDGE SAUCE

168. COCONUT LIME FROSTING

169. CREAMY FROSTING

198. PUMPKIN COOKIES

199. MARSELLAS PANAGOPOULOS BRAZIL NUT ICE CREAM

200. TAHEREH MALEK PUMPKIN ICE CREAM

201. BAKED BROWN RICE

202. GINGER CANDY

203. SANDY MOONEY COFFEE CAKE

204. PAPAYA WALNUT COOKIES

205. LEMON CARROT COOKIES

206. CAROB SANDWICH COOKIES

207. DAISY FROSTING

208. BLACK-EYED PEAS

209. ALMOND BUTTER FROSTING

210. CRUNCH TOPPING FOR ANY BAKED PIE

211. CHERI GILBERT COOKED CAROB GLAZE

212. SUCANANT SUGAR GLAZE

213. ROMA CREAM FROSTING

214. LEMON FILLING

215. BAR-B-QUE SAUCE

216. TOFU FROSTING

217. SWEET SUGAR ICING

218. BLACK EYED IN RICE

219. SOY MILK CORNBREAD

220. OATMEAL ALMOND COOKIE

221. SPICED CUPCAKES

222. DATE OATMEAL COOKIE

223. ORANGE COCONUT COOKIE

224. DATE COOKIE BAR

225. APRICOT COOKIE BAR

226. GINGER PANCAKES

227. LEMON PASTRY

228. LEMON SUGAR COOKIES

229. DATE BROWNIES

230. ORIGINAL SALT WATER TAFFY

231. AURA VICTORIA HUCK PEPPERMINT SALT WATER TAFFY

232. LEMON SALT WATER TAFFY

233. VANILLA SALT WATER TAFFY

234. ORANGE SALT WATER TAFFY

235. JACK PANAGOPOULOS ROMA SALT WATER TAFFY

236. ADRIANA CERRILLO PECAN SALT WATER TAFFY

237. ELMER LYLE MENZIE ALMOND SALT WATER TAFFY

238. ASHLEY SPEIDELL WALNUT SALT WATER TAFFY

239. ROSS H. MENZIE CAROB SALT WATER TAFFY

240. COCONUT SALT WATER TAFFY

241. CINAMMON SALT WATER TAFFY

242. GINGER SALT WATER TAFFY

243. GENE KOENIG ENGLISH TOFFEE CANDY

244. LUCILLE GILBERT LEMON CHEESECAKE

245. ORANGE CHEESECAKE

246. ASHER MICHAEL NEUMILLER CAROB CHEESECAKE

247. ALLIE NICOLE BLUMA NEUMILLER CAROB CAKE

248. DR. EDE VANILLA SUGAR CAKE

249. WALNUT SQUARE COOKIES

250. TARA SHABAFROOZ PECAN SQUARE COOKIES

251. ALMOND SQUARE COOKIES

252. MARGRET ANN MENZIE PECAN ROPE COOKIES

253. MASSOOD SHABAFROOZ WALNUT ROPE COOKIES

254. ALMOND ROPE COOKIES

255. RHI COCONUT OATMEAL CAROB AND ROMA COOKIES

256. RHI COCONUT OATMEAL COOKIES

257. RHI COCONUT OATMEAL WHOLE WHEAT PASTRY FLOUR COOKIES

258. RHI CAROB COCONUT COOKIES

259. RHI COCONUT COOKIES

260. RHI CAROB AND ROMA OATMEAL COOKIES

261. RHI VANILLA DONUTS OR CAKE

262. RHI CAROB BROWN CAKE

263. RHI GOLDEN MACROONS

264. RHI COFFEE MUFFINS

265. RHI SPICED CUP CAKES

266. PEPPERMINT WALNUT FUDGE

267. PEPPERMINT ICE CREAM

268. CAROB AND ROMA ICE CREAM

269. CHERRY FUDGE

270. CAROB ROMA PEPPERMINT ICE CREAM

271. PEACH APRICOT PIE

272. ROMA BAKED ALASKA

273. RAISIN BAR COOKIES

274. FREDERICK HUCK POCKET BREAD FOLDING DIAGRAM

275. NOOSHIN MALEK SEE MOUSEH

276. ZOHREH EHSANI BLUEBERRY ICE CREAM

277. POCKET PIZZA 1

278. RAISIN CREAM PIE

279. DR. EDE KOENIG BEEROCK

280. DATE CREAM PIE

281. POCKET RAISIN PASTRY

282. POCKET PIZZA 3

283. POCKET PIZZA 4

284. POCKET PIZZA 2

285. POCKET DATE PASTRY

286. POCKET PLUM PASTRY

287. PLUM CREAM PIE

288. POCKET CAROB PASTRY

289. POCKET ROMA PASTRY

290. POCKET WALNUT PASTRY

291. POCKET APRICOT PASTRY

292. POCKET CHERRY PASTRY

293. POCKET PEACH PASTRY

294. POCKET PINEAPPLE - LEMON PASTRY

295. POCKET PUMPKIN PASTRY

296. POCKET APPLE PASTRY

297. POCKET EGG ROLLS

298. POCKET BEAN BURRITO

299. APRICOT CREAM PIE

300. VERA WALDSCHMIDT CHERRY CREAM PIE

301. PEACH CREAM PIE

302. APPLE CREAM PIE

303. TAHEREH TAHERIAN HAVANERO HOT SAUCE

304. SHAHNAZ SHAINEE HOT AND SPICY PINTO BEANS

305. PAYAM MALEK ZADEH CAROB WHEAT COOKIES

306. RAISIN ICE CREAM

307. TOMATO CASSEROLE

308. RAISIN FACE COOKIE

309. DATE FACE COOKIE

310. PINEAPPLE COCONUT SQUARES

311. ORANGE PINEAPPLE ICE CREAM

312. LEMON PINEAPPLE ICE CREAM

313. ROMA FACE COOKIE

314. CAROB FACE COOKIE

315. PUMPKIN FACE COOKIE

316. PINEAPPLE FACE COOKIE

317. APPLE FACE COOKIE

318. PEACH FACE COOKIE

319. APRICOT FACE COOKIE

320. PLUM FACE COOKIE

321. CHERRY FACE COOKIE

322. WALNUT DOME COOKIES

323. ALMOND DOME COOKIES

324. PECAN DOME COOKIES

325. CAROB DOME COOKIES

326. ROMA DOME COOKIES

327. COFFEE CUP COOKIE

328. RAISIN CUP COOKIE

329. WALNUT CUP COOKIE

330. POCKET PASTA NO. 4

331. POCKET PASTA NO. 2

332. POCKET PASTA NO. 3

333. POCKET PASTA NO. 1

334. BRAZIL NUT CARMEL CANDY

335. HAVANERO BAKED RICE

336. MACADAMA CARMEL CANDY

337. CINNAMON CARMEL CANDY

338. WALNUT CARMEL CANDY

339. COCONUT CARMEL CANDY

340. PECAN CARMEL CANDY

341. PISTACHIO CARMEL CANDY

342. HAZEL NUT CARMEL CANDY

343. CASHEW CARMEL CANDY

344. ROASTED ALMOND CARMEL CANDY

345. LEMON CARMEL CANDY

346. ORANGE CARMEL CANDY

347. CAROB CARMEL CANDY

348. ROMA CARMEL CANDY

349. PEPPERMINT CARMEL CANDY

350. GINGER CARMEL CANDY

351. HERBS & GARLIC BAKED RICE

352. WALNUT & ALMOND FROSTING

353. PINEAPPLE & LEMON GLAZE

354. ROMA TOFU COOKIES

355. CAROB TOFU COOKIES

356. CINNAMON TOFU COOKIES

357. RAISIN TOFU COOKIES

358. APRICOT TOFU COOKIES

359. DATE TOFU COOKIES

360. CRANBERRIE TOFU COOKIES

361. SPICE TOFU COOKIES

362. PAPAYA TOFU COOKIES

363. COCONUT TOFU COOKIES

364. LEMON TOFU COOKIES

365. ORANGE TOFU COOKIES

366. PINEAPPLE TOFU COOKIES

367. BLACK BEAN SOUP

368. LEMON COCONUT COOKIES

369. CHERRY SUGAR COOKIES

370. ORANGE SUGAR COOKIES

371. RAISIN SUGAR COOKIES

372. ROMA SUGAR COOKIES

373. APPLE SUGAR COOKIES

374. CAROB SUGAR COOKIES

375. PEPPERMINT SUGAR COOKIES

376. BLUEBERRY SUGAR COOKIE

377. DATE SUGAR COOKIE

378. PINEAPPLE SUGAR COOKIE

379. PLUM SUGAR COOKIE

380. PEACH SUGAR COOKIE

381. APRICOT SUGAR COOKIE

382. NECTURINE SUGAR COOKIE

383. CRANBERRY SUGAR COOKIE

384. PUMPKIN SUGAR COOKIE

385. COCONUT CAROB CARMEL CANDY

386. COCONUT LEMON CARMEL CANDY

387. COCONUT CINNAMON CARMEL CANDY

388. COCONUT ORANGE CARMEL CANDY

389. COCONUT PEPPERMINT CARMEL CANDY

390. COCONUT ROMA CARMEL CANDY

391. COCONUT GINGER CARMEL CANY

392. DATE OATMEAL COOKIE

393. RAISIN OATMEAL COOKIE

394. WALNUT DATE COOKIE

395. WALNUT LEMON COOKIE

396. WALNUT RAISIN COOKIE

397. WALNUT ORANGE COOKIE

398. WALNUT CHERRY COOKIE

399. COCONUT DATE COOKIE

400. COCONUT CHERRY COOKIE

401. COCONUT RAISIN COOKIE

402. ONION DRIED ROASTED NUTS

403. GARLIC DRIED ROASTED NUTS

404. HAVANERO DRIED ROASTED NUTS

405. CAYANE DRIED ROASTED NUTS

406. BLACK BEAN RICE

407. SALTED-HAVANERO DRIED ROASTED NUT MIX

408. MAPLE SYRUP DRIED ROASTED NUTS

409. CAROB MACROONS

410. LEMON MACROONS

411. ROMA MACROONS

412. ORANGE MACROONS

413. PEPPERMINT FROSTING

414. PINEAPPLE-LEMON BAKED ALASKA

415. LEMON BAKED ALASKA

416. ORANGE BAKED ALASKA

417. PEPERMINT BAKED ALASKA

418. VANILLA BAKED ALASKA

419. RED HOT FIRE SAUCE

420. APRICOT ICE CREAM

421. TWICE COOKED HERB POTATO

422. PEPPERMINT MACROONS

423. PEACH ICE CREAM

424. TWICE COOKED SPICY POTATO

425. PLUM MACROONS

426. SPICY GARLIC SPREAD

427. ITALIAN SPREAD

428. WALNUT WAFFLES

429. POPPY SEED WAFFLES

430. PUMPKIN SEED WAFFLES

431. CAROB SUCANAT SUGAR COOKIE

432. ROMA SUCANAT SUGAR COOKIE

433. PEPPERMINT SUCANAT SUGAR COOKIE

434. CINNAMON SUCANAT SUGAR COOKIE

435. GINGER SUCANAT SUGAR COOKIE

436. CAROB SUGARED NUTS

437. ROMA SUGARED NUTS

438. PECAN PIE

439. BLUEBERRY CREAM PIE

440. GRAPE PIE

441. LEMON FROSTING

442. ORANGE CAKE FROSTING

443. VANILLA CAKE FROSTING

444. PEACH MAPLE CAKE

445. PLUM MAPLE CAKE

446. APRICOT MAPLE CAKE

447. PINEAPPLE MAPLE CAKE

448. APPLE MAPLE CAKE

449. CHERRY MAPLE CAKE

450. NECTURINE MAPLE CAKE

451. LEMON MAPLE CAKE

452. ORANGE MAPLE CAKE

453. BLUEBERRY MAPLE CAKE

454. PEAR MAPLE CAKE

455. BLUEBERRY BAKED ALASKA

456. BAR- B- QUE HOT SAUCE

457. PISTACHIO WAFFELS

458. PEACH BAKED ALASKA

459. APRICOT BAKED ALASKA

460. APPLE BAKED ALASKA

461. PLUM BAKED ALASKA

462. NECTURINE BAKED ALASKA

463. GRAPE BAKED ALASKA

464. CHEESE SAUCE FOR BAKED POTATO

465. APPLE ICE CREAM

466. PLUM ICE CREAM

467. GRAPE ICE CREAM

468. PEAR ICE CREAM

469. RHI MAPLE SYRUP COOKIES

470. MAPLE SYRUP BROWNIES

471. CAROB NUGGET CANDY

472. ROMA NUGGET CANDY

473. PEPPERMINT NUGGET CANDY

474. CINNAMON NUGGET CANDY

475. LEMON NUGGET CANDY

476. VANILLA NUGGET CANDY

477. APRICOT NUGGET CANDY

478. ITALIAN DRY ROASTED NUT MIX

479. GARLIC DRY ROASTED PUFF CORN MIX

480. ONION DRY ROASTED PUFF CORN MIX

481. HAVENARO DRY ROASTED PUFF CORN MIX

482. CAYENNE DRY ROASTED PUFF CORN MIX

483. ITALIAN DRY ROASTED PUFF CORN MIX

484. SALTED DRY ROASTED PUFF CORN MIX

485. CAJUN DRY ROASTED PUFF CORN MIX

486. SALTED HAVENARO DRY ROASTED PUFF C ORN MIX

487. PLUM TOFU COOKIES

488. PEACH TOFU COOKIES

489. NECTARINE TOFU COOKIES

490. SPICY AVACADO DIP

491. ALL PURPOSE GRAVY

492. POTATO AND CABBAGE STEW

493. CAROB PIE CRUST

494. ROMA PIE CRUST

495. COFFEE BAKED PIE

496. CRANBERRY SAUCE

497. GREEN BEANS CASSAROLE

498. QUICK OATMEAL

499. BAKED YAMS

500. SAUTE CORN

501. CINNAMON AND GINGER COOKIES

502. ORANGE NUGGET CANDY

503. POTATO AND CELERY SOUP

504. AVACADO DIP

505. CARROT SOUP

506. PEACH UPSIDE DOWN CREAM CAKE

507. APRICOT UPSIDE DOWN CREAM CAKE

508. NECTARINE UPSIDE DOWN CREAM CAKE

509. CHERRY UPSIDE DOWN CREAM CAKE

510. GRAPE UPSIDE DOWN CREAM CAKE

511. APPLE UPSIDE DOWN CREAM CAKE

512. CINNAMON UPSIDE DOWN CREAM CAKE

513. CAROB UPSIDE DOWN CREAM CAKE

514. PLUM UPSOIDE DOWN CREAM CAKE

515. ROMA UPSIDE DOWN CREAM CAKE

516. PINEAPPLE UPSIDE DOWN CREAM CAKE

517. PEPPERMINT UPSIDE DOWN CREAM CAKE

518. ORANGE UPSIDE DOWN CREAM CAKE

519. LEMON UPSIDE DOWN CREAM CAKE

520. GINGER UPSIDE DOWN CREAM CAKE

521. JAMACIAN RICE

522. LEMON AND OLIVE BASMATI RICE MIX

523. CARROT AND OLIVE BASMATI RICE MIX

524. GARLIC AND ONION SAUTED CORN

525. GREEN JALAPENO RICE MIX

526. ROASTED PISTACHIO CANDY

527. PISTACHIO FUDGE

528. SPICY CORN BREAD

529. RED HOT ROAST

530. CINNAMON WALNUT COOKIES

531. ORANGE BALL COOKIES

532. LEMON BALL COOKIES

533. ORANGE PASTRY

534. CINNAMON MACROONS

535. CINNAMON AND OATMEAL COOKIES

536. RED POTATO CASSEROLE

537. CINNAMON ICE CREAM

538. DATE WALNUT TART

539. WALNUT GINGER COOKIES

540. WALNUT ROMA COOKIES

541. WALNUT CAROB COOKIES

542. SLICE WALNUT COOKIES

543. LEMON AND HERB DRY ROASTED NUT MIX

544. LEMON AND DILL DRY ROASTED NUT MIX

545. LEMON AND SALTED DRY ROASTED NUT MIX

546. SWEET AND SOUR DRY ROASTED NUT MIX

547. LEMON AND CAYANNE DRY ROASTED NUT MIX

548. LEMON AND CAJON DRY ROASTED NUT MIX

549. LEMON AND HAVENERO ROASTED NUT MIX

550. LEMON AND ONION DRY ROASTED NUT MIX

Ingredients To Avoid

Bha-butylated bht hydroytolune
Black Strap Molasses
Caffeine
Calcium Sulfate
Carmel
Carrageen
Disodium Sulfite
Distilled water - (do not use- no minerals)
Edtacalcium disodium
Ethylenediamine
Letracetate
Gum Arabic
Cellulose chatti karaya
Gypsum
Hydroylated lecithin
Monocalcium Satisfactory Phosphate
Hydrolyzed protein
Lactic Acid
Magnesium chlorate
Maltodextrim - white sugar
Magnesium Sterate
Modified food starch
Mono+dislycerides
Mono sodium glutamate
M S G
Multol dextrin
Natural flavor
Nisarl
Non hydroxylated Lecithin
Phosforic acid
Popylgallate
Propylene Glycolalginate

Polysorbate 60, 65, 80
Red Dye 40 - Allura Red AC
Stearic Acid
Sodium Saccharin
Sodium Alginate
Sodium Benzoate
Sodium Bicarbonate
Sodium Chloride
Sodium Erythrobate
Sulfur Dioxide
Sugar black paperbicarbonate of soda
Tragacanth Xanthan
Torutein
Vinegar
Yeast flakes

References

Ede Koenig MD., Founder and Director of the Radiant Health Institute

Michel Klaper MD., Director of the Institute of Nutrition, Education, and Research

Sidney M Whittaker MD.

Monroe Rosenthal MD.

Medical, Pritican

Agatha Thrash

Milton G Crane MD.

James Dobson MD.

M.Beddow Bayly MD.

John McDougal MD.

John Harvey Kellogg MD.

Raymond Moore MD.

Kari F Meyer MD.

Owen S Parrett MD.

About the Author

For almost the past ten years understanding health has been very interesting, and I have applied this information to improve my life. I have and will continue to inspire others who want to do the same. I give away thousands of food items yearly and encourage others to share their food. I develop and research food recipes, adding to my approximate 600 recipes to date. I have won 55 awards for my cooking, in addition, have written eight books on health and cooking. All books include recipes, which work in concert with a healthy body. Most of all I continue to maintain a healthy life style and I am an example of what good food and a clean body can accomplish. As I share this information, I hope to show how easy this completely healthy life style is to achieve. These benefits are incredible, and not limited to only a few. I will never go backto a life of pain and suffering and declining health. There is just no legitimate reason to not maintain a healthy life style through good nutrition and avoidance of all drugs.

Science cannot replace nature and cannot fool the body. In the long term, the body will malfunction if not treated properly. I can say for certain that to continue abusing the body and maintaining disease with drugs does not make any sense. Research done on drugs in the United States shows that good health and drugs are not related, but to avoid sickness through proper nutrition will guarantee good health and are closely related.